WOLFF-PARKISON-WHITE SYNDROME

INTO THE PROCEEDURES FOR HEALING WOLFF-PARKISON-WHITE SYNDROME

DR. AHMED .R

Contents

CHAPTER ONE

INTRODUCTION

A tachycardia, or rapid heartbeat, is brought on by an additional electrical pathway that runs between the ventricles and atria of your heart in Wolff-Parkinson-White (WPW) syndrome.

The additional electrical route is rather uncommon and present from birth. Approximately 4 out of every 100,000 individuals have WPW. The symptoms associated with Wolff-Parkinson-White syndrome can affect people of all ages, even newborns. Most symptomatic individuals initially notice symptoms between the ages of 11 and 50.

Fast heartbeat events are normally not fatal, although they can lead to major cardiac issues. Treatment for Wolff-Parkinson-White syndrome can halt or avoid heart-pounding episodes. Ablation is a catheter-based technique that can permanently fix irregular heart rhythms.

Symptoms

A rapid heartbeat is the cause of Wolff-Parkinson-White syndrome symptoms. People in their teens or 20s are more likely to experience them for the first time. The following are typical signs of WPW syndrome:

Palpitations are the sensation of fast, fluttering, or pounding heartbeats.

lightheadedness

dizziness

Losing consciousness

Easily being tired when working out

Uncertainty

A quick start to an episode of rapid heartbeat might last anywhere from a few seconds to several hours. Exercise is a common trigger for episodes. For some people, alcohol and caffeine or other stimulants might act as triggers. Up to 25% of persons with WPW may eventually no longer feel their symptoms.

A form of abnormal heartbeat known as atrial fibrillation is occasionally experienced by 10 to 30 percent of individuals with Wolff-Parkinson-White syndrome. Among the WPW symptoms and indicators in these individuals are:

chest ache

tightness in the chest

breathing difficulties

Occasionally, unexpected death

Infants' symptoms

Infants with Wolff-Parkinson-White syndrome may exhibit the following symptoms:

Breathlessness

Absence of activity or alertness

Bad cuisine

palpable fast heartbeats in the chest

Absence of symptoms

The majority of persons with an additional electrical route in their hearts do not have symptoms or a rapid heartbeat. The Wolff-Parkinson-White pattern is a disorder that is only incidentally found during a patient's routine cardiac checkup. For many individuals, the Wolff-Parkinson-White pattern is benign. However, physicians could advise additional testing prior to high-intensity sports participation for kids with WPW patterns.

When to visit a physician

Heart irregularities, or arrhythmias, can be caused by a variety of illnesses. It's critical to receive appropriate care and a timely, correct diagnosis. If you or your kid exhibits any symptoms related to Wolff-Parkinson-White syndrome, make an appointment with your physician.

If you suffer any of the following symptoms for longer than a few minutes, call 911 or your local emergency number:

accelerated or erratic heart rate

breathing difficulties

chest ache

Reasons

A tachycardia, or rapid heartbeat, is brought on by an additional electrical pathway that runs between the ventricles and atria of your heart in Wolff-Parkinson-White (WPW) syndrome. The Wolff-Parkinson-White syndrome pathway is present from birth. In a tiny number of cases, the syndrome is caused by an aberrant gene (gene mutation). Additionally, congenital cardiac diseases like Ebstein's abnormality are linked to WPW. Elsewise, little is understood regarding the development of this additional pathway.

typical electrical circuit of the heart

There are two upper chambers (called atria) and two lower chambers (called ventricles) that make up your heart. Normally, a mass of tissue in the right atrium called the sinus node regulates the rhythm of your heart. Every heartbeat is produced by electrical impulses that come from the sinus node.

Muscle contractions brought on by these electrical impulses pass through the atria and pump blood into the ventricles. The atrioventricular node (AV node), a group of cells that receives the electrical impulses, is typically the only channel via which signals can pass from the atria to the ventricles. Prior to sending the electrical signal to the ventricles, the AV node slows it down. The ventricles can fill with blood thanks to this small delay. Muscle contractions allow electrical impulses to enter the ventricles, which then pump blood to the lungs and other parts of the body.

WPW's unusual electrical system

An additional electrical channel that links the ventricles and atria permits electrical impulses to avoid the AV node in Wolff-Parkinson-White syndrome. This diversion of the electrical impulses through the heart causes pre-excitation, or premature activation of the ventricles.

The additional electrical channel may result in one of two main kinds of rhythm abnormalities:

electrical impulses looped. The electrical impulses from the heart travel up one channel after traveling down the extra or regular one in WPW, forming a full electrical loop of signals. This disorder, known as AV reentrant tachycardia, causes the ventricles to receive impulses very quickly. Consequently, the ventricles pump rapidly, resulting in a rapid heartbeat.

electrical impulses that are not well structured. The atria may beat rapidly and irregularly (atrial fibrillation) if electrical impulses start in the wrong place in the right atrium and spread across the atria in an unorganized manner. The ventricles may beat more quickly as a result of the disordered signals and the additional WPW route. Consequently, the ventricles are unable to fill with blood in time, resulting in insufficient blood flow to the body.

COMMITMENTS

Wolff-Parkinson-White syndrome doesn't usually result in serious issues for most people. However, issues can arise, and it's not always easy to determine your risk of experiencing life-threatening cardiac episodes. In example, if you have other cardiac issues, you may suffer the following if the disorder remains untreated:

Periods of fainting (syncope)

accelerated heart rate (tachycardia)

Occasionally, unexpected death

CHAPTER TWO

Getting Ready for Your Consultation

You will probably be referred to a heart specialist (cardiologist) whether you see your family doctor first or receive emergency care. Here are some tips to help you prepare for your visit and understand what to anticipate from your physician.

What you're capable of

Jot down all of your symptoms, even if they don't seem to have anything to do with your heart.

Enumerate all of your prescription drugs, vitamins, and dietary supplements.

Jot down your vital signs and any additional conditions that have been diagnosed.

Important details about you, such as any recent changes or stresses in your life, should be put in writing.

Questions to put to your physician

Which of my symptoms is most likely to be the cause?

Which tests are necessary for me?

Which medical procedures are beneficial?

Which dangers are associated with my heart condition?

How often are follow-up appointments required?

Do I have to limit what I do?

What effect will my drugs or other illnesses I have on my heart problem?

Don't be afraid to ask questions during your appointment, in addition to the ones you have prepared for your doctor.

What to anticipate from your physician

You'll probably be asked a lot of questions by your doctor. Being prepared to respond to them could free up time to discuss topics you'd like to spend more time on. One may ask you:

How severe are your symptoms, and when did you start feeling them?

How frequently has your heartbeat been rapid?

What is the duration of the episodes?

Does anything seem to set off or exacerbate the episodes, such as stress, exercise, or caffeine?

Does heart disease run in your family?

Exams and diagnosis

A physical examination, a health history, and lab tests such as the following are likely to be performed by your doctor first:

Tests on your blood to measure potassium and thyroid hormone levels, which might cause some cardiac rhythm problems.

X-ray of the chest to see if your heart is enlarged.

Your doctor will then probably suggest cardiac testing.

An ECG

Small sensors called electrodes are affixed to your arms and chest during an electrocardiogram (ECG) to record electrical signals as they pass through your heart. Your physician can examine these signals for patterns that point to the existence of an additional electrical route in your heart. Even if you're not having an episode of rapid heartbeat right now, this pathway can typically be identified.

In order to get more details regarding your heart rate, your doctor might also advise you to use portable ECG equipment at home. Among these gadgets are:

Holter observation. You can wear this compact ECG gadget on a belt or shoulder strap, or carry it in your pocket. It gives your doctor a longer look at your heart rhythms by recording your heart's activity for a full day. Most likely, during the course of the day, your doctor will urge you to keep a journal in which you will describe any symptoms you feel and note when they happen.

Recorder of events. Over the course of a few weeks to several months, your heart activity will be monitored by this portable ECG gadget. The recorder is only turned on when you are experiencing symptoms of an elevated heart rate.

Testing using electrophysiology

This test can be utilized to identify the additional pathway's location or to confirm a diagnosis of Wolff-Parkinson-White syndrome. You will typically be given medicine to help you relax while you are awake. Electrodes are inserted into thin, flexible tubes called catheters and threaded through your blood veins to different locations within your heart. The electrodes can locate an additional electrical channel and accurately track the distribution of electrical impulses throughout each beat once they are in situ.

MEDICATIONS AND SUBTLES

The severity and frequency of your symptoms are just two of the variables that determine how you will be treated.

You most likely won't require treatment if you have the Wolff-Parkinson-White pathway but don't exhibit any symptoms. If therapy is required, the objective is to stop an episode of rapid heartbeat and to slow down similar events in the future. Among the choices are:

Vagal techniques. Coughing, putting an ice pack on your face, and bearing down as though you are having a bowel movement are examples of basic physical actions that affect the vagus nerve, which helps control your heartbeat. If your heartbeat becomes too fast, your doctor could advise you to use vagal movements to help slow it down.

Drugs. You could require an injection of an anti-arrhythmic drug if vagal exercises are ineffective in halting the rapid heartbeat. Additionally, your doctor might suggest a medicine that lowers heart rate.

a cardioversion. To assist your heart return to a regular rhythm, your doctor could apply paddles or patches to your chest. When therapies and pills don't work, cardioversion is usually employed.

Ablation of a catheter using radiofrequency. Your heart is reached by thin, flexible tubes called catheters that are inserted into blood arteries. The additional electrical route causing your illness is destroyed (ablated) by heating the electrodes at the tips of the catheters. Up to 95% of patients with Wolff-Parkinson-White syndrome respond well to radiofrequency ablation.

It's likely that your doctor may advise follow-up visits to check on the rhythm and rate of your heart.

THE END